Sex

Kama Sutra

Top 20 Sex Positions

by

Anna Shine

Table of Contents

Introduction

I would like to thank you for purchasing the book, " SEX: KAMA SUTRA - Top 20 Sex Positions".

Sex is one of the most beautiful things in the world, but it can become pretty boring if you keep doing the same thing over and over again. The sad thing is that most people usually don't know exactly what to do to bring that spark back into the bedroom.

Are you tired of the same old missionary sex position? Do you want to find different ways to spice up your sex life? Are you looking for something to help you look forward to sex with excitement? If you do, then you are in the right place.

This book brings you 20 best sex positions you can try today and be glad you did plus tips on how to spice up your sex life and tantric massage techniques.

Thanks again for purchasing this book, I hope you enjoy it!

7 Sensual Secrets To Being A Tantric Lover

1. Breathe in more deeply: When with your partner, take in deeper breaths. Breathing deeply into your groin, belly and your chest will awaken all your sensual charisma and this awakened sensual charisma will be felt by your partner, which will turn him/her on.

2. Gaze into your partner's eyes: This is yet another very simple technique, but only a few people get to look into other people's eyes eventually. On the first date, you may look into your partner or potential lover's eyes out of curiosity, then familiarity sets in making you forget that you still have a lot to learn about your partner. There is something really juicy about taking a time to stare into the eyes of your partner and allowing them look into yours at the same time. It is a telepathic way of telling your partner that you are not scared of letting them to see you and they have all your attention at that moment. An important thing to note as you do this is to ensure that the stare is natural and intimate without trying to be creepy about the stare. Over time, your partner will see you only want to connect with him/her, which will heat things up between you two.

3. Listen to what your partner's body is saying: Your partner's body speaks too. The body has several ways of letting you know if it is a yes or a no from your partner at any point in time. Things like a crossed arm show your partner is afraid and on the defensive, a woman running her fingers through her hair means she wants you, if he/she touches you playfully, it shows your partner or potential lover want it there and then. Following these cues will help you know what your partner wants. If you are not sure, you can ask them what they want in a sexy whisper.

4. Feather light touch: Once you get the permission to get closer, begin with the slightest and slowest feather light touch you can manage to come up with. The lighter your touch, the greater the sensation your touch will create on your partner and the more the arousal. You can increase the firmness and speed of your touch. However, make sure you start with the slow, sensual strokes and return to them later to ensure your partner stays aroused with all his/her sensuality awakened for as long as the intimacy lasts.

5. Take things a little bit slow: It is fun to have a hard and fast lovemaking session, but if you don't change things occasionally, things will definitely become desensitizing and robotic. To master the act of Tantric sex techniques, you need to slow down your pace, practice prolonging the pleasure time and delay the satisfaction for as long as possible. Add up all the aforementioned steps to this and you will find a deeper connection with your partner for the most passionate lovemaking.

6. Spread some sexual energy: You can follow your breath while using coconut oil to massage your partner's chest/breast and rib cage. You can also get your lover to breathe in a slower, deeper pace. Run your fingers from your partner's sexual center and move up to the stomach, between the chest/breast, over the throat, lips, and then caress through his/her hair and then exhale the energy down his/her legs and all the way to their feet. You can then work your way up to the innermost part of their thighs, and give their sex organ a tantalizing touch. Repeat this procedure and pay attention to the movement of their body whenever you touch a particular spot. The main aim here is to spread the sexual pleasure all over your partner's body. Spreading sexual energy this way starts a sexual ripple throughout every inch of your partner's body helping him/her hit multiple orgasms. This works for both sexes.

7. Breast message: The breasts are no doubt an intimacy center. Think about it this way. Your heart sits close to your breasts. Your heart is much more than a physical pump that helps keep you alive; it also serves as the place where you feel the deepest emotions, love, and connection.

When your breasts are stimulated with gentle pinches, the love and bonding hormone known as oxytocin is released. In women, this action causes the lifting of the cervix and uterus, making them more prepared for penetration. A sensual breast massage can arouse both a man and a woman. Always remember to switch to the gentle caresses after stimulating the breasts and listen to what your partner wants often.

5 Yoni Massage Techniques To Tickle Your Woman

Once you have succeeded in warming up your partner's body with nipple stimulation and breast massage, it is now time to move on to the yoni massage as the man.

1. Circling

Circle the tip of your woman's clitoris with the tip of your finger to arouse your partner. The circling could vary from smaller circles to larger circles. You can alternate the pressure from mild, to intense.

2. Pushing and pulling

Push down on the woman's clitoris and make some little push and pull strokes before sliding your finger down the clitoris shaft. However, always remember that some women show more sensitivity on one part of the clitoris than others do.

3. Tugging and rolling

To tug your woman's clitoris, gently pull the clit away from the body by grasping its sides and tugging at it back and forth. You could equally move lower and tug the lips of the clitoris while varying strokes from the top of the clitoris to its lips. In order to roll your woman's clitoris, begin by holding firmly and roll between the index finger and the thumb as if making a tiny violin stroke using your fingers.

4. Tapping

Making use of one or more fingers, tap your woman's clitoris in different rhythms beginning from fast and moving to slow to enable you to learn what her body responds to the most.

5. G-spot massage

To discover the G-spot, keep your first two fingers in a curved position to resemble the letter C and slide the curved fingers into the vagina. Once there, feel for a piece of skin with a spongy feel behind the woman's clitoris. Massage that point by moving your curved fingers back and forth. Use varying strokes from fast to slow. You can simultaneously tickle the clitoris at the tip while at it.

Best Kneeling Sex Positions

Who said you have to lie down to have sex. Below are amazing ways to have sex while kneeling

1. The Kneeling sex position

The kneeling fox sex position is great for deep penetration.

How the kneeling sex position works

For the woman: Get down on your hands and knees and lean forward on both arms.

For the man: Kneel, then grab hold of her waist and enter her from behind.

The pros

For the man: Men love the doggy-style position, so this is bound to be an exciting experience for you.

The cons

Since you won't be able to look at each other, it means you won't be able to kiss during sex, which reduces the intimacy.

2. The melody maker

The melody maker sex position is great for achieving fast mind blowing orgasm.

How the melody maker sex position works

This sex position is a little bit more tricky than others and you will need a footstool or a comfortable chair.

For the woman: Sit on the chair sideways, lean backwards and keep your head pointing downwards.

For the man: Kneel between her legs and enter her. It is advisable that you hold hands to give the woman some support.

The pros

For the woman: Having your head pointing in a downwards position will make you get an amazing rush of blood, especially by the time you hit orgasm.

The cons

This sex position might feel a little bit odd at first and it might be difficult for you to maintain that position for a long time.

3. Hit the G-spot

The hit the spot sex position is great for hitting the woman's G-spot.

How the hit the spot sex position works

For the woman: Lie down on your stomach with your hips swiveling sideways and your legs bent.

For the man: Kneel between the woman's legs and lean forward with your arms on either side of the woman. You can now thrust.

The pros

For the woman: As can be seen from the name, this position helps you get amazing G-spot orgasms.

The cons

For the woman: You might not enjoy not being able to look at your man's face while, since you are facing down.

Best Standing Sex Positions

Having sex while standing is an amazing way to not only enjoy sex but also to burn more calories. Below are some amazing standing sex positions you can try out:

4. Standing up

This sex position is appropriate for hitting the woman's G-spot easily and faster.

How the standing up sex position works

For the woman: Stand while facing the wall, about two feet away from the man and stick your bum out slightly.

For the man: Penetrate and ensure you bend your knees, as this helps you enter the woman more easily and deeply.

The pros

With this sex position, you can thrust backwards which is much easier than most other sex positions that require you to sit down.

The turn-offs

You just have to stand up for this one, which is a possible turn off for some people because it calls for more effort than most other sex positions.

5. The Manhandle Her

This sex position is great for pleasuring the woman as the man pleasures her by touching her in the right places.

How the manhandle her sex position works

You won't need a bed for this one-you can do it anywhere around your house such as the bathroom, kitchen, bedroom, living room, etc. But you might need to be close to a wall for some balance.

For the woman: Stand in front of the man and bend a little forward, and then straighten up slowly, as the man's penis remains in your love garden. If you find it a bit awkward, you can continue leaning forward, which makes it easy for him to continue holding on to you. You don't need to do much after that other than leaning back and enjoying yourself.

For the man: When the two of you are ready, you can start thrusting slowly at first, then harder.

The cons

This position is great for achieving amazing orgasm from different stimulation areas. For instance, the man can rub the woman's clitoris and breast at the same time.

The cons

This position can make it a bit hard for the woman to maintain her balance.

Best Sitting Sex Positions

There are also some amazing sex positions that you can try while seated.

6. Edge of Heaven

This sex position is great for helping the woman orgasm faster.

How the edge of heaven sex position works

For the man: Sit down on the edge of a bed or chair with your legs on the floor. Hold the woman's hands to ensure she doesn't tip backwards.

For the woman: Move on to the man's lap, with your legs resting on the bed or stretched at the back of the chair. Move slowly or fast depending on your speed preferences.

The pros

The woman gets very deep penetrations while the man does most of the work.

The cons

The woman might tip over if she is not careful.

7. Face to face

This sensuous sex position is great for some simple but exciting sex after a hectic day at work.

How the face-to-face sex position works

For the man: Put your feet together in order to provide some type of cradle for the woman.

For the woman: Sit down opposite the man, then slide into the man's lap and sit down on top of him, and then join your legs behind the man. Simply rock on the man continuously.

The pros

The face-to-face sex position helps you both reach orgasm at the same time because the two of you build up sexual energy until you both reach climax.

The cons

Some people may find this sex position slow and tame.

Best Man On Top Sex Positions

Below are some amazing sex positions that enable the man to take control.

8. The man trap

This sex position is great for orgasmic week-night sex, especially when there is very little energy to go all the way. The man trap position is one sex position that comes quite close to replacing the age-long missionary style sex position.

How the man trap sex position works

For the woman: Simply lie on the bed on your back. Once the man lies on you, you wrap your legs around his legs. Wrapping your legs around him gives you some kind of control to control his speed and the rhythm. Arch your back a little bit to enjoy the benefits of this sex position.

For the man: Get on top of the woman, and thrust in and out while her legs are wrapped around yours.

The pros

For the woman: You will get a powerful orgasm from the feeling of his body rubbing against yours.

For the man: You get aroused by her legs entwining around you.

9. Speed Bump

This sex position is great for having fast and passionate sex.

How the speed bump sex position works

For the woman: Lie flat on your stomach with a pillow under the pelvic and stomach area, then spread your legs.

For the man: Lie on top of her and penetrate her.

The pros

This is one great sex position for those fast and furious quickies.

The cons

The skin-to-skin contact can make you sweaty which is not so appealing to most people.

Best Woman On Top Sex Positions

10. Woman on top

The sex position is great for both of you because you get pleasured at the same rate.

How this sex position works

For the man: Lie down on the bed with your two legs stretched out in front of you.

For the woman: Climb on top the man like some cowgirl while the man penetrates you. You can then lean on your back and hold onto the man's knees and ankles if he raises them up. From then you can control the pace and tease the man occasionally.

The pros

The man will definitely love this because he has a great view while you enjoy it because you are the one in charge here.

The cons

The woman does all the work.

11. The Sultry Saddle

This sex position is known to be great for couples who have been looking for something new to try during sex.

How it works

For the man: Lie down and keep your knees and legs wide apart.

For the woman: Slot into the middle at a right-angled position to the man's body. With one of your hands on the man's chest, and the other hand on the man's lower leg. Starts rocking back and forth gently at first, then adding more momentum gradually.

The pros

You can control how things go with this style by wiggling around until everything feels all right.

The cons

You might have to practice a while before things start feeling right with this sex position. It might feel awkward at first, but you don't have to worry about that because you will love it after a while.

Generally, this sex position might slow down the pace of your sex for a while, but in the end, the fun justifies the effort you put into mastering the sultry paddle.

12. The Squat

This sex position is great for you because it sure promises you the most sensational sexual experience.

How the squat sex position works

For the man: Simply lie down on your back on the bed while facing up. To pleasure the woman while on it, you can caress her breasts using both hands.

For the woman: Squat right on top of the man. That's all there is to the squat sex position. Then gently raise yourself up and down on the man. You can increase your speed with time to increase the fun and sensation.

The pros

This sex position helps you get stimulated far more than you anticipated

The cons

The woman might tip forward is she doesn't take adequate care, and this could be painful for the man.

13. Reverse cowgirl

This sex position is great for hitting the woman's magic G-spot. This sex position is a kind of a cross between the doggy-style and the classic woman on top position.

How the reverse cowgirl sex position works

For the man: Lie on your back on the bed.

For the woman: Climb on top of your man while facing away from him and lean forward with your palms resting on his thighs or knees. Angle his penis a little downward while he enters you. Rock back and forth for that unforgettable, G-spot hitting sensation.

The pros

For the woman: You control the angle, movement, and speed, and this position gives you a great view if you love watching yourself in the mirror having sex.

The cons

There will be minimal physical contact between the two of you.

14. Corridor Canoodling

This sex position is great for afternoon quickies.

How the corridor Canoodling sex position works

Find a part of your home where two opposite walls are close to each other such as a corridor or bathroom.

For the man: Lean against one wall and shuffle down so you could be in a sitting position with your back on one wall and your feet pushed against the opposite wall.

For the woman: Climb on top of him with his legs supporting your entire weight while your feet dangle from both sides. You then thrust back and forth on top of him like you would in a sitting position.

The pros

This position is perfect for a spontaneous and exciting sexual experience when you two just have to have it quickly.

The cons

He will need to have enough stamina on his legs to carry your weight and it could take you a while to get used to this position.

15. Galloping Horse

The galloping horse sex position is great for the both of you.

How the galloping horse sex position works

For the man: Sit on a comfortable chair with your legs stretched out in front of you.

For the woman: Climb onto your man and stretch your legs out straight behind him, lean back while holding to him for support while he clings. You are in control here, so push back and forth on top of him as fast as you wish for as long as you like.

The pros

For the man: You get a good view

For the woman: You get a good penetration.

The cons

For the woman: It might be a bit uncomfortable for you to keep your legs stretched out for a long time.

16. The Good Spread

The good spread sex position is great for the woman as she is the one on the driver's seat.

How the good spread sex position works

For the man: Lie down flat on your back.

For the woman: Climb on top of your man and start spreading out your legs slowly as far as you can spread them. Then place your two hands on his chest and rock back and forth.

The pros

For the woman: The wider apart you can spread your legs, the deeper the penetration you get, which is great for both of you.

The cons

For the woman: The stretch on your legs can start hurting after a while.

Best Lying Down Sex Positions

17. The Scissors

This sex position is just great for the most intimate sex.

How the scissors sex position works

This one can be said to be easy to do, yet hard to explain. The way to go about this sex position is to lie down while facing each other.

For the woman: Place your top leg across the man's hip.

For the man: Grab the woman's bum and place your arms around her waist and push her bottom leg against your leg.

The pros

This position enables the woman to rub her clitoral area on the man's groin while the two keep kissing.

The cons

Some may find this a little bit boring and pedestrian.

18. The Spider

This sex position is most appropriate for a long slow sexual experience.

How the spider sex position works

For the woman: Lie down on your back, and put your legs in-between your man's legs.

For the man: Follow suit until your two legs enclose the woman's.

Then each of you can raise your knees up and hold onto each other's legs. Now, all you have to do is keep wiggling with very slow movements to make sure you keep each other sexually aroused for long.

The pros

This can be a very lazy sex position in case you love it hot and fast. However, it is an enjoyable sex position that can help keep you happy for long.

The cons

There are quite a few actions and movements, which most people might find boring.

19. Spooning

This sex position is great for slow, intimate sex.

How the sexy spoons sex position works

For the woman: Lie down on the bed on your side.

For the man: Spoon her from behind, entering her slowly to make the bedtime cuddle a more exciting experience.

The pros

This sex position helps you two feel intimate and close, and helps you and your partner get a very amazing orgasm.

The cons

This sex position might appear a bit awkward at first, but if you stick to it, it will definitely become an important part of your sex regimen.

20. The magic bullet

The magic bullet sex position is another great sex position for hitting the woman's G-spot.

How the magic bullet sex position works

For the woman: Lie face up on the bed while straightening your legs up in the air.

For the man: Kneel on the bed behind the woman, hold on to her legs for thrusts and leverage.

The pros

For the man: You can push up her legs with one hand while touching her anywhere you like with the other hand.

The cons

For the woman: Your legs can start feeling achy after a while.

The Best Ways To Spice Up Your Sex Life

Leaning about the 20 most exciting sex positions is never going to be enough to make your sex life a very exciting one unless you learn how to make things a little bit more spicy and sensational. It is not just about engaging in the most romantic sex positions, it is also important that you learn how to put your partner in the mood at all times. Sometimes it is not the sex itself that makes the whole thing very exciting, the foreplay also plays a great role in ensuring things get very sensational and hot. Here are a collection of tips and techniques you can rely on to help you make things more exciting and get your partner in the right mood for sex anytime:

For The Woman

Say YES to Sex

Before you talk about making things more exciting in your sex life with your partner, you must say yes to sex by embracing it and giving it all you have. This means you have to be more open to sex and sexual ideas from your partner. Saying yes to sex implies doing all in your power to engage in sex as often as possible without using the common excuses women use such as, "I had a hectic day at work and can't have sex right now", "I'm simply not in the mood", "I have a serious headache", and all other such lines you might want to use to deny your partner sex.

Initiate sex more often

Another great way to spice up your sex life is to be the one to make the move more often. Don't make the mistake of believing that the task of initiating sex is solely a man's role. Anyone can initiate the sex, and it becomes sexier if you do so more often. It even gets better if you two get into some kind of competition as to who initiates sex more, which makes you have twice as much sex.

Go lacy

Believe it or not, nothing turns the man on when you remove your clothes than the sight of those lacy undies. Be it panties or bra, the lacier they are, the sexier the man will find you. Always wear sexy underwear and some nice lingerie to get your man in the mood. Nothing makes someone get out of the mood than unattractive underwear.

Wear red

Men agree that there is something quite sexy and almost irresistible about a woman in red. If you can get more red panties, the sight of them will help turn your man on the more. You can get a mix of white and red, pink, purple, and all other such bright colors to brighten things up a little more.

Get more colorful interior decor for your bedroom

If you want him to find the room sexier when he gets home or the next time he visits, try laying a red bedspread. Other beautiful colors you can include are pink and purple. You can equally get flowers and other accessories in these sexy colors for the bedroom.

Flirt with him

If you want him to want you more often, learn to flirt with him more often. Flirting with your man makes him feel wanted and nothing drives a man crazy than knowing that you do want him.

For The Man

There are several ways you can spice up your sex life as the man. Here are some ways you can make things more exciting in your marriage or relationship:

Tell her how sexy she looks

Women put in a lot of effort trying to look sexy and attractive, and as the man, it is your duty to compliment her efforts often. When she goes shopping for new undies or dresses just to look good for you, make sure you tell her how sexy she looks. Women are moved by words so do well to let her know she looks sexy as often as possible.

Ensure you spend a considerable amount of time on foreplay

Most men make the mistake of jumping into sex after a few kisses, but this is not going to help spice things up in your sex life. Take more time to kiss her most erogenous zones such as her ears, her nape, her navel, breasts, and pubic area. Kiss and touch your woman in the right places and take some time enjoying each others caresses before moving on to having sex.

Be adventurous

Don't let things get mundane in your sex life. Find ways to try out some new styles and sex position. You can read books, search the internet or watch videos of exciting sex positions and styles you can try out with your partner.

Exercise more

Nothing kills the passion in your sex life with your partner more than your inability to get your sex tool to rise up to the occasion when the need arises. Engaging in more physical exercises will not only help you become more energetic and gain stamina, but will go a long way in helping you take care of common sexual problems like erectile dysfunction. Physical exercises will help you last longer during sex, which makes it the more exciting.

Engage in more morning sex

Studies have found out that men are able to perform better when they have sex in the morning and last longer because testosterone levels peak in the morning, which helps them last longer. In addition, morning sex has been found to improve your mood.

48

Thank you!

Love,

Anna Shine

Printed in Great Britain
by Amazon

46586631R00030